HOW TO STOP NEGATIVE THOUGHTS

A comprehensive guide in letting go of negative thoughts

Daniel L. Wilson 2022

Table of Contents

CHAPTER ONE

What are Negative Thoughts?

Can you identify with the sentiments described below?

I sometimes find myself pondering specifically over a bad situation

A terrifying expectation of what's going to happen next or in the future usually keeps me busy

There is always an unstated desire to be affirmed by my loved ones to feel secure and satisfied with myself and my choices

I tend to feel depressed, unhappy, frustrated, and cranky when things do not go my way

Often, I find myself expecting a lot from people/ loved ones and when they fail to deliver, I cling onto it against them and myself too

I doubt myself someplace even though I know the other person has done me wrong

I simply find positives to not be very persuasive or realistic based on my observation and experiences in life

We may be able to connect to some of these concepts with varying degrees of intensity.

Never-ending negative thoughts frequently make the issue greater than it is in our minds, therefore depriving us of our peace of mind and pleasure. Such mental processes create an easy prescription for negative thinking, which drags individuals into despair, anxiety, and poor self-worth. When pressured with a barrage of such negative ideas, we start to question whether there is a more effective approach to conquering them. Many motivational speakers and self-help publications believe that positive thinking is a choice, but it never seems that straightforward.

Definition of Negative Thoughts:
"Negative thoughts are cognitions about the self, others, or the environment in general that are characterized by negative perceptions, expectancies, and attributions that are related

with unpleasant feelings and bad behavioral, physiological, and health outcomes."

The negative thought description from Rethink Mental Illness indicates that:

"Negative thought refers to a tendency of thinking destructively about yourself and your environment. While everyone experiences negative thoughts very often, negative thinking that seriously affects the way you think about yourself and the world and even interferes with work/study and everyday functioning could be a symptom of a mental illness, including depression, anxiety disorders, and personality disorders"

Negative thoughts - Origin and Types:
The genesis of negative thoughts is often founded on the negative basic beliefs that we hold about ourselves and the way we perceive the world. Learning is dependent on observation and experience and when growing up if both

have influenced a person badly then they tend to absorb and execute that.

For example: If you were continually compared to someone while growing up; you tend to become more critical of yourself.

If you observed your parents not enjoying a wonderful connection, there is most probable potential that you could wind up questioning your relationship.

If you've experienced infidelity, the prospect of creating a meaningful relationship again feels like a job.

It's as if our unpleasant experiences and observations start influencing the way we should act rather than being our real selves. It's fairly normal however it's feasible to have a better knowledge of our cognition to not hang onto these negative beliefs. It's crucial to know and examine what might be the probable cognitive mistakes that make us feel and think this way to attempt and overcome them.

Cognitive mistakes are erroneous notions that could impact your emotions. Everyone encounters these mistakes to some level yet their more severe versions may be distressful for a person. The checklist of these errors is:

All-or-nothing thinking: We see things either in black or white categories. There is less or no space for a grey area to exist that makes things polarised.
If we do not do our best, we perceive ourselves as a complete failure.

Overgeneralization: We regard a single bad incident as a never-ending pattern of loss so construct wide interpretations out of a single event.

Mental filter: We choose to choose a single negative feature and linger on it all together that distorts our perspective of reality exactly like

like a drop of ink that discolors the whole beaker of water.

Disqualifying the good: We fail to embrace pleasant experiences by declaring they 'don't count for some reason or other. In this manner, we wind up holding a negative viewpoint that is countered by our daily experiences.
One could have a nice day but yet chooses to focus on the one unpleasant thing that occurred.

Jumping to conclusions: Making negative inferences and assumptions without having a clear fact that firmly back our findings.
She doesn't pay me enough attention ergo she doesn't love me.

Mind reading: Interpreting the thoughts ad beliefs of another without appropriate proof. She would not go on a date with me. She undoubtedly thinks I'm foolish.

Fortune Telling: We are confident that our prognosis is an established reality and based on it we foresee that things will turn out terribly Magnification (catastrophizing) or minimization: When we either exaggerate our mistakes or flaws (Magnification) or are indifferent towards our or other people's strengths and positives (Minimisation) (Minimisation).

Emotional reasoning: When we go by the saying, I feel it, therefore it must be true. It is the ritual of making decisions based on how we feel rather than being objective. We assume that our undesirable emotions or feelings define the reality of how things are, when in practicality they may be different.

Should statements: We attempt to motivate/reprimand ourselves with 'should' and 'shouldn't', 'musts', and 'ought to have. The emotional effects are guilt. 'Should' remarks when directed toward others would make you feel angry, upset, and worried.

Labeling: This is an extreme kind of over-generalization. One applies a negative label to oneself - "I'm a nasty person" instead of expressing our mistake, when someone else's action touches us the wrong way, we ascribe a negative name to that person. He lied to me ergo all guys are liars.

Personalization: It is a mistake when a person feels that everything others do or say is some type of a direct, unique response towards them. They take things personally, even even if it is not intended in that manner.

CHAPTER TWO

Causes of Negative thoughts

We all have bad ideas at times. Anger, anxiety, humiliation, and other unpleasant feelings are natural when they occur and then pass away. However, if you become locked in negative thinking patterns, not only can they make you sad, but they may also induce or aggravate anxiety and depression and can even have a detrimental influence on things like your immune system and your health.

Identify Causes of Negative Thinking
Negative thinking may take various forms. The most prevalent reasons for negative thinking are the following:

Overanalyzing and Indecisiveness
When making significant choices, it is vital to take your time and evaluate your alternatives. However, examining the options might turn into

obsessing over them. Set a deadline for the decision. Allow yourself a decent amount of time for study and contemplation, but then make your decision and stick to it.

Negative Rumination About Past Events

A certain level of thought about where you have been and how it influences your life now is beneficial. But when those ideas become negative and you spend too much time on them, that thinking pattern may be harmful. To cease ruminating on the past, concentrate on the present by taking up a new activity, passion, or task. Doing so may help put prior difficulties into their appropriate perspective.

Outward-directed Anger

We have all been mistreated by someone, whether a family member, friend or stranger. In some cases, these experiences cause us to have a negative opinion not only of that person but everyone like him or her or people in general. Negative feelings like these can cause us to lash out or withdraw. A healthier approach when you are consumed by anger at someone is to try and see the world from his or her point of view. This can bring better understanding and help you see others in a new, less negative light.

Fear of the Future

The future is unknown to us and can be a source of anxiety. In some people, this leads to the bad habit of always assuming that the worse is yet to come. This is unrealistic and also a waste of emotional energy. You can limit the impact of negative thinking about the future by accepting that we have only limited control over it and keying in on those factors that we do control.

Negative Self-criticism

Excessive self-criticism can also be a source of negative thinking. Although it is important, to be honest with yourself about your strengths and weaknesses, negative self-criticism, if taken to extremes, can reduce your confidence in your ability to tackle life's challenges. Strive for a balanced perspective of your character and achievements, rather than continually accentuating the bad.

Lack of self-confidence

A lack of self-confidence is directly tied to being too critical of oneself. To build your confidence, remind yourself of what you accomplished well, rather than concentrating entirely on the bad. Be careful to give yourself credit for the excellent things you have accomplished. You might also try obtaining a new viewpoint by asking a loved one what he or she thinks. You could be pleasantly surprised with the reaction.

Jumping to Conclusions

Another sort of negative thinking is leaping conclusions about what other people think about you. Assuming the worst in their eyes is often a misunderstanding of what they truly believe, which could be more insightful and complex than you know. If you are doubtful, ask the individual in question. An honest remark may eliminate ambiguity and help clear the air.

Self-blame

It is crucial to assume responsibility for the choices we make over circumstances that we control. But taking on undue responsibility for those occurrences that are out of our control might have a bad influence on our life. We don't carry the weight of the world on our shoulders, only those little spaces in which we live, love, and work.

Catastrophizing

Catastrophizing is the mental habit of always assuming the worst possible outcome in any situation, even when more realistic possibilities exist. Some people 'catastrophize' as a hedge against feeling upset or disappointed if something doesn't go their way. Catastrophizing is closely connected to dread of the future and should be fought similarly.

Lack of self-confidence

A lack of self-confidence is directly tied to being too critical of oneself. To build your confidence, remind yourself of what you accomplished well, rather than concentrating entirely on the bad. Be careful to give yourself credit for the excellent things you have accomplished. You might also try obtaining a new viewpoint by asking a loved one what he or she thinks. You could be pleasantly surprised with the reaction.

Labeling

Labels are basic assessments that we pass on ourselves, frequently to negative effect. After an emotional breakup, someone can claim, "I'm simply no good at relationships." That sentiment might be used to rationalize a lack of effort in future relationships. The defeatism of this sort is another form of pessimistic thinking.

Negative Thoughts Will Trigger Negative Emotions

Negative thinking doesn't exist without repercussions. It may influence every element of your life, including how you feel, your relationships with others, and the quality of your decision-making. Negative thinking may even influence your health, wearing down your immune and other biological systems via continuous stress and heightened levels of worry. Hypertension, recurrent infections, digestive diseases, and cardiovascular disease have all been related to prolonged stress.

Mental Health Disorders That Intensify Negative Thinking

Negative thinking may have numerous origins, including personal reasons such as enduring a terrible event. That said, scientists are finding evidence that certain mental health disorders play a critical role in the habitual formation of dark or negative thoughts. Researchers have identified three conditions in particular that often have an impact.

Obsessive-compulsive Disorder (OCD)

A third mental health problem underpinning negative thinking is obsessive-compulsive disorder OCD. This disorder is characterized as the recurring experience of intrusive and unwelcome thoughts, that force a person to irresistibly execute specific (often monotonous and unproductive) chores to avert some injury or accident. These routine behaviors can be debilitating because they interfere with the normal conduct of life. OCD can generate negative thoughts similar to depression, but these tend to be more blatantly irrational than those associated with the latter.

Generalized Anxiety Disorder (GAD)

Generalized Anxiety Disorder, or GAD, is another possible antecedent to negative thinking. Persons with GAD suffer a constant sense of worry and anxiety about every area of their life, even when things seem to be going well. This may lead to the mental habits of dreading the future and catastrophizing, which we've previously highlighted as indications of negative thinking.

Depression

Depression is a mental health illness defined by apparently inevitable emotions of melancholy, lethargy, pessimism, and a fatalistic view of one's future. Associated with it are physical symptoms such as a lack of energy, decreased appetite, longer-than-normal sleep periods, loss of focus, and, in rare instances, acts of self-harm. The link between depression and negative thinking is established.

CHAPTER THREE

Effects of Negative thoughts

We all have an inner critic. At times this tiny voice may be beneficial and keep us driven toward goals—like when it warns us that what we're going to eat isn't healthy or that what we're about to do may not be prudent. However, this voice may frequently be more damaging than beneficial, especially when it falls into the area of extreme negativity. This is known as negative thoughts, and it can knock us down.

Negative thoughts is something that most of us encounter from time to time, and it comes in various forms. It also produces enormous stress, not just to ourselves but to everyone around us if we're not cautious. Here's everything you need to know about negative thoughts and its consequences on your body, your mind, your life, and your loved ones.

Negative thoughts may take various forms. It might seem grounded ("I'm not good at this, therefore I should avoid doing it for my safety," for example) or it's simply cruel ("I can never do anything well!"). It may look like a fair evaluation of a circumstance ("I got a C on this exam. I suppose I'm not good at arithmetic."), only to deteriorate into a fear-based fantasy ("I'll never be able to go to a decent college").

The reflections of your inner critic may sound a lot like a judgmental parent or friend from your past. It may follow the course of common cognitive distortions: catastrophizing, blaming, and the like.

Consequences of Negative thoughts

Negative thoughts may influence us in some fairly detrimental ways. One large-scale investigation indicated that rumination and self-blame about unfavorable occurrences were connected to an increased risk of mental health problems.

Focusing on negative thoughts may lead to decreased motivation as well as greater feelings of helplessness. This type of critical inner dialogue has even been linked to depression, so it's something to fix.

Those who find themselves constantly indulging in negative thoughts are likely to be more anxious. This is in large part because their reality is changed to create an experience where they can't attain the objectives they've set for themselves.

Negative thoughts may lead to a lessened capacity to identify possibilities, as well as a decreased likelihood to capitalize on these chances. This implies that the heightened experience of stress arises from both the perception and the changes in behavior that occur from it. Other implications of negative thoughts might include:

Limited thinking: The more you tell yourself you can't accomplish something, the more you believe it.

Perfectionism: You come to sincerely think that "excellent" isn't as good as "perfect," and that perfection is possible. In contrast, simple high performers tend to fare better than their perfectionistic counterparts since they are typically less stressed and are content with a job well done. They don't tear it apart and attempt to home in on what might have been better.

Symptoms of depression: Some studies have indicated that negative thoughts may lead to a worsening of feelings of depression. If left uncontrolled, this might be highly detrimental.

Relationship challenges: Whether the continual self-criticism makes you look needy and insecure or you transfer your negative thoughts into more general bad behaviors that affect others, a lack of communication and even a "playful" amount of criticism may take a toll.

One of the most apparent problems of negative thoughts is that it's not positive. This seems basic, yet research has proven that positive thoughts is a strong predictor of success.

For example, one study on athletes compared four different types of thoughts (instructional, motivational, positive, and negative) and found that positive thoughts was the greatest predictor of success. People didn't need to remind themselves how to do something as much as they needed to tell themselves that they are doing something great and that others notice it as well.

How to Minimize Negative thoughts
There are many ways to reduce thoughts in your daily life. Different tactics work better for different individuals, so try a few and find which ones are most beneficial for you.

Catch Your Critic
Learn to detect when you're being self-critical so you can begin to quit. For example, observe

when you say things to yourself that you wouldn't say to a close friend or a kid.

Remember That Thoughts and Feelings Aren't Always Reality

Thinking bad things about oneself may seem like keen observations, but your ideas and emotions about yourself can not be regarded as facts. Your ideas may be warped like everyone else's, vulnerable to prejudices and the effect of your emotions.

Give Your Inner Critic a Nickname

There was once a "Saturday Night Live" character known as Debbie Downer. She would find the bad in every scenario. If your inner critic has this questionable ability as well, you might tell yourself, "Debbie Downer is doing her thing again."

When you conceive of your inner critic as a force outside of yourself and even give it a silly moniker, it's not just more simple to recognize that you don't have to agree, but it becomes less scary and easier to see how ludicrous some of your critical ideas may be.

Contain Your Negativity

If you find yourself participating in negative thoughts, it helps to restrict the harm that a critical inner voice may create by just allowing it to criticize select items in your life, or be negative for only an hour in your day. This puts a limit on how much negativity can come from the situation.

Change Negativity to Neutrality

When engaged in negative thoughts, you may be able to catch yourself, but it may often be tough to push yourself to halt a train of thinking in its tracks. It's generally considerably simpler to modify the intensity of your words. "I can't tolerate this" becomes, "This is tough." "I despise..." becomes, "I don't like..." and even, "I don't prefer..." When your thoughts utilizes more soothing language, much of its negative impact is subdued as well.

Cross-Examine Your Inner Critic

One of the destructive characteristics of negative thoughts is that it typically goes unchecked. After all, if it's going on in your brain, people may not be aware of what you're saying and therefore can't tell you how incorrect you are.

It's a lot better to notice your negative thoughts and question how accurate it is. The great majority of negative thoughts is an exaggeration, and calling yourself on this may help to take away its destructive impact.

Think Like a Friend

When our inner critic is at its worst, it might sound like our deadliest adversary. Often we'll say things to ourselves in our minds that we'd never say to a buddy. Why not reverse this and—when you catch yourself speaking negatively in your head—make it a point to imagine yourself saying this to a treasured friend?

If you know you wouldn't say it this way, think of how you'd share your thoughts with a good friend or what you'd like a good friend to say to you. This is a great way to shift your thoughts in general.

Shift Your Perspective

Sometimes looking at things, in the long run, might enable you to see that you may be putting too large a focus on something. For example, you may ask yourself whether anything you're outraged over will truly matter in five years or even one.

Another technique to adjust perspective is to pretend that you are panning out and looking at your issues from a vast distance. Even thinking of the world as a globe and of yourself as a little, tiny individual on this globe might remind you that most of your troubles aren't as huge as they appear. This may typically lessen the negativity, dread, and urgency in negative thoughts.

Even tossing certain negative thoughts words around under your breath might remind you how absurd and impractical they seem. This will remind you to give yourself a break.

Stop That Thought

For others, merely stopping negative ideas in their tracks might be therapeutic. This is known as "thought-stopping" and might take the form of snapping a rubber band around your wrist, imagining a stop sign, or just moving to another idea when a negative one enters your head. This may be useful with recurrent or excessively critical thoughts such as, "I'm no good," or, "I'll never be able to accomplish this," for example.

Replace the Bad With Some Good

This is one of the finest methods of countering negative thoughts: Replace it with something better. Take a negative notion and replace it with something uplifting that's equally truthful.

Repeat until you find yourself needing to do it less and less often. This works well with most bad habits: replacing unhealthy food with healthy food, for example. It's a terrific method to build a more optimistic way of thinking about yourself and life.

CHAPTER FOUR

Getting rid of negative thoughts

To have negative thoughts is to be human and the fight against negativity may sometimes be weight-heavy. This is precisely why you may continuously question yourself about how to get rid of negative thoughts. Well, you'd be astonished to find the solution to this question is a lot more straightforward than it looks.

Even the simplest things might quickly drown behind the loudness and relentless avalanche of negative ideas that appear justified. If you could ignore that noise, what would you do?

Make new acquaintances or explore a new career? It isn't that you have a mind full of over-eager negative notions.

Our mind is constantly on red alert to talk with a negative voice. Here are methods to understand why negative thoughts are highly damaging and how to cope with them.

13 Ways to Get Rid of Negative Thoughts
Check out these go-to ways to send negative thoughts on their merry way.

1. Identify the Triggers
As you learn to examine your thoughts without judgment, try to seek patterns in these spirals from a distance. Is there a common trigger point that kickstarts this spiral? And once you recognize that, don't stop there.

Dig deeper to understand the triggers and the underlying emotions behind them. What about the trigger genuinely impacting you so much? Are there unaddressed difficulties hiding underneath there? Instead of fixing the symptoms, consider if you can address the main problem.

If it is too emotionally weighty, go to a therapist to sort things out together. Healing those open wounds or bruised scars below could assist resolve these spirals in the long term.

2. Read It Out

There has been a tendency for celebrities to read their bad social media messages out loud, and when you witness that you understand how stupid and ludicrous they are. Try it out with the negative voice within your brain. Call up a buddy, share your bad ideas with them, and then laugh at how stupid the mind can be.

By repeating these words out loud, you will shift the energy surrounding it, and it will be easier for you to let go of the negative thinking and replace it with something good. You'll be astonished at how this suggestion on how to cope with negative thoughts might improve your life.

3. Tell a Joke or Funny Story

Laughter always brings you to a better perspective. Smile, tell a joke, or remember a funny story. Laughing at yourself can never be a bad thing either! Laughter does wonders to the spirit - it's a terrific passion that makes your life better because you become happier and healthier.

When you feel negative thoughts start to seep in, remember that you can always counteract them with this advice. Of course, that doesn't imply you have to make a joke about everything. It simply implies that doing something that makes you laugh or smile is the greatest method to overcome negative thoughts.

4. Speak Back

Negative ideas appreciate being in power. When it tries to take over, do what I do. Mentally say to it, "thanks for sharing," and continue with your day. There is no point battling with it since it will become louder. Just speak back to it and move on!

It takes conscious effort to follow this tip. When you sense negative thoughts start seeping in, catch yourself. This awareness will guarantee you can talk back and convert the notion into something different. For example, if you put on a dress and you start thinking badly about yourself, take a deep breath and look in the mirror. Instead of belittling yourself, reassure yourself that you are confident and you look good.

5. Breathe

Calm your mind by taking three deep breaths. Stop what you are doing, get your feet linked with the earth, and breathe deeply. Don't hurry them, breathe in and out, and consider your next action.

Breathing does wonders for the mind. This is why it's a vital aspect of meditation. Breathe in and out, and feel the oxygen fill your body up from your nose to your lungs. Breath-based meditation may also be done by quietly counting your inhalations and exhalations so you can concentrate on them instead of your bothersome thoughts.

The key to breathing as a type of meditation is simply awareness. After practicing this technique, notice whether you can feel your body start to relax.

6. Set a Time-Limit

Hanging around with your bad ideas won't help them go away. Tell yourself that you will accept such ideas for no more than one minute and then they are no longer welcome. For an extra incentive, put a timer on your smartphone. Once it turns off, don't let any bad ideas back in.

This concrete technique on how to get rid of negative thoughts is one even novices can follow effortlessly. After all, you can't immediately shut out negative ideas the instant it begins seeping in.

By conducting a countdown, you may examine your negative thoughts and prepare yourself for them. You can't just "turn off" your mind, but you may slow it down to a tolerable level by cutting out superfluous chatter.

7. Exercise

Exercise helps ease your mood and the current boom in group exercise mind/body sessions underscores that. This makes it one of the most crucial strategies in how to erase negative thoughts.

Smart fitness fans have been doing this for years by taking the breakthrough mind-body workout, IntenSati, where you educate your mind to say happy ideas and employ the intents from class in your daily life. One popular sentence spoken out loud in class goes like this, "all negative thoughts halt right now! "

Through exercises like IntenSati, you can turn daily exercise from something that used to be mindless drudgery into something that is not only life-affirming but also excellent for your mind and body.

This training strategy may even boost your cognitive and psychological function.

Moreover, it may do wonders to help you feel fantastic about yourself, and in time, it will make you recognize the value of living a life that you enjoy.

8. Change Your Environment
Learning how to rid your mind of negative ideas is no simple thing. However, a change of surroundings, simply stepping out of the room you are in, may transfer the mind to different thinking patterns.

Stand up and move away from the situation and find something fresh to concentrate on. You may look at folding the clothes from a whole new, and more pleasant perspective.

For example, if you are hanging out in your room and you're beginning to hear negative ideas in your head, walk outside the home and open your window. If you want to go the additional mile, you may stroll around your neighborhood. Doing this will provide you access to new items to alter your emphasis.

Following this suggestion may even help you look at folding the clothes from a whole new, and more pleasant perspective.

9. Write It Down

Negativity kills positivity so get those thoughts out of your head. Set a timer for 5 to 10 minutes and jot down all your anxieties. Once you have done this, crumple up the sheet of paper, shred it up, and toss away that list. Get it off your chest and move on.

Writing does wonders for our capacity to think clearly and rationally, and you let your anxieties out. It provides you an opportunity to look at yourself from a new perspective and obtain some type of strength. This is particularly beneficial when you're trying to go ahead with anything.

10. Use Affirmations

Do you want to know how to stop negative thoughts? Prepare a positive remark to say to yourself when negative thinking occurs. For example, "yes I can, I can do it, I am in the process of finding it out." Find one that speaks to you and keep it on hand to fight off the negative voice.

It doesn't have to be a whole sentence. Sometimes, it might simply be one word or a phrase that communicates what you want to tell yourself. Repeat it over and again in your head until you feel the bad ideas depart.

Saying affirmations is a terrific technique to start the morning in a good and light tone before permitting any negative ideas to come through.

11. Use a Go-to Mannerism

Have fun with this one. When a negative thought appears, react with a fun or silly action. Poke your tongue out, slap your wrist, or just smile. Find a physiological reaction that will bring you out of your thoughts and concentrate back on the present. This advice might help you learn how to stop spinning.

By linking your attempt to avoid unpleasant thoughts with an action, you may concentrate more on the response instead of the idea itself. The concept which accompanies the bad emotion just disappears into the background.

12. Observe Without Judgment

When we start going down the spiral of negative thinking, we are generally our toughest critics. "How foolish was I not to see this coming? " "How could I even think this was possible? " "What is wrong with me? " "I keep making the same mistakes." "Won't I ever learn my lesson? "

The next time you find yourself swimming in the deep end with such negative ideas, try to transfer to the seat of the observer. See if you can rise above the thoughts and observe from a distance. Often, when we are too close to the situation, we fail to see how our thoughts are nonsensical or ridiculous.

Becoming an observer is like holding up the mirror to reflect on our cognitive processes. This honest and non-judgmental introspection helps us identify the errors in our cognitive processes. We start seeing and perceiving the things we were blinded to while we were in the thick of things, and it helps us go ahead.

13. Stop Comparing Yourself to Others

This is a huge tip in learning how to get free from negative thoughts. It's incredibly easy to compare yourself to other people in today's social media environment. Research indicated that the more time individuals spend on Facebook, the more miserable they are.

People like to communicate their successes through status updates and publish favorable images. It's tempting to compare yourself to your friends' Facebook façade and come up wanting. Then, you decide to publish an update that makes you appear nice, and if it doesn't receive a ton of likes and comments, you get the feeling your Facebook friends don't like you.

This applies a great lot to those who are in relationships as well. Oftentimes, they do so because they've seen their friends do the same. If you're not in a happy relationship, seeing someone's favorable status in the artificial atmosphere of social media may be a severe downer. You find yourself comparing yourself to them without even realizing it.

Final Thoughts
The tips shared above should have answered the ringing question of how to get rid of negative thoughts. Remember, the mind is a vital and holy area. Keep things clean and transparent.

Whenever you feel yourself sliding down this rabbit hole of negative thoughts, anchor yourself intentionally to the present moment. Bring your consciousness to your current reality and watch the ideas from a distance. Remind yourself that you are much more than your ideas and emotions.

CHAPTER FIVE

Regulating your thoughts

How to Control Your Thoughts and Be the Master of Your Mind is the most powerful instrument you have for the production of the good in your life, but if not utilized appropriately, can also be the most destructive force in your life. To manage your ideas is to impact the way you conduct your life.

Your mind, more particularly, your ideas, impacts your perception and consequently, your interpretation of reality. (And Here's Why Your Perception Is Your Reality)

I have heard that the typical human thinks roughly 70,000 thoughts a day. That's a lot, particularly if they are unproductive, self-abusive, and simply a general waste of energy.

You may let your ideas run crazy, but why would you? It is your mind, your ideas; isn't it time to reclaim your control back? Isn't it time to take control?

Choose to be the person who is actively, knowingly thinking about your ideas. Be someone who can manage your thoughts—become the master of your mind.

When you alter your thinking, you will change your emotions as well, and you will also remove the triggers that set off those sensations. Both of these results give you a better amount of calm in your mind.

I presently have a few ideas that are neither of my choice nor a reaction to my reprogramming. I am the ruler of my thoughts, thus now my mind is fairly serene. Yours can be too!

Before you can become the master of your mind, you must acknowledge that you are presently at the mercy of numerous undesirable "squatters" dwelling in your mind, and they are in charge of your ideas.

If you want to be their boss, you must know who they are and what their objective is, and then you can take command and evict them.

Here are four of the "squatters" in your brain that cause harmful and unproductive ideas.

1. The Inner Critic

This is your continuous abuser who is generally a mixture of:

Other people's words—many times your parents
Thoughts you have developed based on your own or other peoples' expectations
Comparing oneself to other people, even those in the media
The thoughts you tell yourself as a consequence of terrible situations such as betrayal and rejection. Your perception causes your self-doubt and self-blame, which are most frequently unfair in circumstances of rejection and betrayal.

The Inner Critic is driven by suffering, poor self-esteem, lack of self-acceptance, and lack of self-love.

Why else would this individual assault you? And because this person is you—why else would you mistreat yourself? Why would you let someone treat you this badly?

2. The Warrior

This individual lives in the future—in the realm of "what ifs."

The Warrior is driven by dread, which is frequently illogical and has no substance. Occasionally, this individual is driven by a dread that what occurred in the past will happen again.

3. The Reactor or Troublemaker

This is the one that produces rage, irritation, and suffering. These triggers arise from unhealed wounds of the past. Any incident that is even loosely similar to a former hurt can send him off.

This individual may be set off by words or sentiments and can also be set off by noises and odors.

The Reactor has no true drive and weak impulse control. He is governed by old programming that no longer helps you—if it ever did.

4. The Sleep Deprived
This may be a mix of any number of distinct squatters including the inner planner, the rehashing, and the ruminator, along with the inner critic and the worrier.

The Sleep Depriver's motive might be:

As a response to quiet, which he fights against
Taking care of the business you ignored throughout the day
Self-doubt, poor self-esteem, insecurity, and generalized anxiety
As noted above the inner critic and worrier
How do you handle these squatters?

How to Master Your Mind

You are the thinker and the spectator of your ideas. You can manage your thoughts, but you must pay attention to them so you can identify "who" is directing the show—this will define which approach you will wish to apply.

Begin each day to pay attention to your thoughts and catch yourself when you are thinking negative ideas.

There are two techniques to manage your thoughts:

Technique A – Interrupt and replace them
Technique B – Eliminate them completely
This second alternative is what is known as peace of mind.

The approach of interrupting and replacing is a strategy for changing your subconscious mind. Eventually, the replacement thoughts will become the "go-to" thoughts in applicable situations.

Use Technique A with the Inner Critic and Worrier and Technique B with the Reactor and Sleep Deprived.

1. For the Inner Critic
When you notice yourself thinking anything bad about yourself (calling yourself names, demeaning yourself, or berating yourself), stop it.

You may shout (in your head), "Stop! No! " alternatively, "Enough! I'm in charge now." Then, whatever your negative idea was about yourself, replace it with an opposing or counterthought or an affirmation that starts with "I am."

For example, if your thinking is, "I'm such a loser," you might replace it with, "I am a Divine Creation of the Universal Spirit. I am a perfect spiritual entity learning to conquer the earthly experience. I am a being of energy, light, and matter. I am great, intelligent, and gorgeous. I adore and approve of myself exactly as I am."

You may also hold a debate with yourself to refute the 'voice' that formed the thought—if you know whose voice it is:

"Just because so-and-so claimed I was a loser doesn't make it true. It was his or her opinion, not a declaration of truth. Or maybe they were kidding and I took it seriously because I'm insecure."

If you know that you have frequent self-critical thoughts, you may write down or pre-plan your counter ideas or affirmation so you can be ready.

This is the first squatter you should evict, forcibly, if necessary:

They rile up the Worrier.

The names you call yourself become triggers when called such names by others, thus he also retains the existence of the Reactor.

They are typically there when you attempt to fall asleep thus he maintains the Sleep Deprived.

They are a bully and are verbally and emotionally abusive.

They are the destroyer of self-esteem. They convince you that you're not worthy. They're liars! For the sake of your self-worth, get them out!

Eliminate your harshest critic and you will also lessen the presence of the other three squatters.

Replace them with your new best friends that support, encourage, and enrich your life. This is a presence you desire in your head.

2. For the Worrier

Prolonged anxiety is mentally, emotionally, and physically unhealthy. It may have long-term health repercussions.

Fear begins the fight or flight reaction, produces concern in the mind, and creates anxiety in the body. This may make it more difficult for you to regulate your thoughts efficiently.

You should be able to spot a "worry thought" quickly by how you feel. The physiological signals that the fight or flight reaction of terror has set in are:

Increased heart rate, blood pressure, or burst of adrenaline
Shallow breathing or breathlessness
Muscles tighten
Use the above-stated strategy to interrupt any thought of anxiety and then replace it. But this time, you will replace your thoughts of concern with feelings of thankfulness for the result you want.

If you believe in a higher power, now is the moment to interact with it. Here is an example:

Instead of worrying about my loved ones traveling in bad weather, I say the following (I call it a prayer):

"Thank you in great spirits for watching over me. Thank you for watching over his/her car and keeping it safe, road-worthy, and free of maintenance issues without warning. Thank you for surrounding him/her with only safe, diligent, and aware drivers. And thank you for keeping him/her safe, conscientious, and alert."

Smile when you think about it or say it aloud, and phrase it in the present tense. Both of these will help you feel it and possibly even start to believe it.

If you can envision what you are praying for, the visualization will heighten the sensation thus you will boost the influence in your vibrational field.

Now, take a calming breath, slowly in through your nose, and slowly out through the mouth.

Take as many as you like! Do it until you feel that you're close to being in control of your thoughts.

Replacing scared thoughts with appreciation will minimize reactive behavior, taking the steam out of the Reactor.

For example: If your kid gets lost at the mall, the traditional parental response that follows the scared feelings while finding them is to scold them.

"I told you never to leave my sight." This reply merely adds to the child's worry level from being lost in the first place.

Plus, it also teaches them that mom and/or dad will get furious when he or she makes a mistake, which may make them lie to you or not tell you things in the future.

Change those fearful thoughts when they happen:

"Thank You (your choice of Higher Power) for watching over my child and keeping him safe. Thank you for helping me locate him soon."

Then, when you see your child after this thought process, your only reaction will be gratitude, and that seems like a better alternative for all people involved.

3. For the Troublemaker, Reactor or Over-Reactor

Permanently eradicating this squatter will need a little more focus and contemplation after the event to discover and cure the sources of the triggers. But until then, you may keep the Reactor from getting out of hand by commencing mindful breathing as soon as you notice his existence.

The Reactor's thoughts or feelings activate the fight or flight response just like with the Worrier. The physiological signs of his presence will be the same. With a little attention, you should be able to tell the difference between anxiety, anger, frustration, or pain.

I'm sure you've heard the suggestion to count to ten when you get angry—well, you can make those ten seconds much more productive if you are breathing consciously during that time.

Mindful breathing is as easy as it sounds—just be conscious of your breathing. Pay attention to the air moving in and coming out.

Breathe in via your nose:
Feel the air entering your nostrils.
Feel your lungs full and expanding.
Focus on your belly rising.

Breathe out through your nose:
Feel your lungs emptying.
Focus on your belly falling.
Feel the air exiting your nostrils.

Do this for as long as you like. Leave the situation if you want. This gives the adrenaline time to normalize. Now, you can address the situation with a calmer, more rational perspective and avoid damaging behavior, and you'll be more in control of your thoughts.

One of the complications this squatter brings is that it adds to the sleep depriver's concerns. By evicting or at least controlling the Reactor, you will decrease reactionary behavior, which will decrease the need for the rehashing and ruminating that may keep you from falling asleep.

Master your thoughts and stop the Reactor from generating stress for you and your relationships!

Most importantly, find your real motive. What's the inner motivation that might allow you to keep on moving? If you're not sure, join the free Fast-Track Class – Activate Your Motivation. It's a free intense session that will help you find your inner drive and develop your motivation engine around it. Join the free session here.

4. For the Sleep Deprived

(They're made up of the Inner Planner, the Rehasher, and the Ruminator, along with the Inner Critic and the Worrier.)

I was troubled with a fairly frequent problem: not being able to turn off my thoughts at sleep. This limitation hindered me from falling asleep and consequently, having a comfortable and restorative night's sleep.

Here's how I disciplined my thoughts and banished the Sleep Depriver and all his pals.

I began by concentrating on my breathing—paying attention to the rise and fall of my belly—but it didn't keep the ideas out for long. (Actually, I now start with examining my at-rest mouth posture to prevent me from clenching.)
Then I came up with a new approach that removed uncontrolled thinking—imagining the word in when breathing in and thinking the word out while breathing out. I would (and do)

elongate the word to match the length of my breath.

When I catch myself thinking, I shift back to in, out. With this technique, I am still thinking, sort of, but the wheels are no longer spinning out of control. I am in control of my mind and thoughts, and I choose quiet.

From the first time I tried this method, I started to yawn after only a few cycles and am usually asleep within ten minutes.

For really difficult nights, I add increased attention by holding my eyes in a looking-up position (closed, of course) (closed, of course). Sometimes I try to look toward my third eye but that hurts my eyes.

If you have trouble falling asleep because you can't shut off your mind, I strongly recommend you try this technique. I still use it every night. You can start sleeping better tonight!

You may also use this strategy each time you wish to:

- Fall back to sleep if you wake up too soon
- Shut down your thinking
- Calm your emotions
- Simply focus on the present moment.

The Bottom Line

Your mind is a tool, and like any other tool, it can be used for constructive purposes or destructive purposes.

You can allow your mind to be occupied by unwanted, undesirable, and destructive tenants, or you can choose desirable tenants like peace, gratitude, compassion, love, and joy.

Your mind can become your best friend, your biggest supporter, and someone you can count on to be there and encourage you. You can be in control of your thoughts. The option is yours!

www.ingramcontent.com/pod-product-compliance
Lightning Source LLC
Chambersburg PA
CBHW071551260726
48653CB00007BA/2777